Living With Lung Cancer

Strategies for Wellness and Living a Fulfilling Life

Rossana Lewis

TABLE OF CONTENT

Chapter 1: Understanding Lung Cancer

Lung cancer is a disease caused by uncontrolled cell division in your lungs. Your cells divide and make more copies of themselves as a part of their normal function. But sometimes, they get changes (mutations) that cause them to keep making more of themselves when they shouldn't. Damaged cells dividing uncontrollably create masses, or tumors, of tissue that eventually keep your organs from working properly. This cancer is the name for cancers that start in your lungs — usually in the airways (bronchi or bronchioles) or small air sacs (alveoli). Cancers that start in other places and move to your lungs are usually named for where they start (your healthcare provider may refer to this as cancer that's metastatic to your lungs). It is the third most common cancer in the US.

1.1 Types and Stages of Lung Cancer

There are many cancers that affect the lungs, but we usually use the term "lung cancer" for two main kinds: non-small cell lung cancer and small cell lung cancer.

Non-small cell lung cancer (NSCLC) is the most common type of lung cancer. It accounts for over 80% of lung cancer cases. Common types include adenocarcinoma and squamous cell carcinoma. Adenosquamous carcinoma and sarcomatoid carcinoma are two less common types of NSCLC.

Small cell lung cancer (SCLC) grows more quickly and is harder to treat than NSCLC. It's often found as a relatively small lung tumor that's already spread to other parts of your body. Specific types of SCLC include small cell carcinoma (also called oat cell carcinoma) and combined small cell carcinoma.

Other types of cancer can start in or around your lungs, including lymphomas (cancer in your lymph nodes), sarcomas (cancer in your bones or soft tissue) and pleural mesothelioma (cancer in the lining of your lungs). These are treated differently and usually aren't referred to as lung cancer.

What are the Stages of Lung Cancer?
Cancer is usually staged based on the size of the initial tumor, how far or deep into the

surrounding tissue it goes, and whether it's spread to lymph nodes or other organs. Each type of cancer has its own guidelines for staging.

Each stage has several combinations of size and spread that can fall into that category. For instance, the primary tumor in a Stage III cancer could be smaller than in a Stage II cancer, but other factors put it at a more advanced stage. The general staging for lung cancer is:

Stage 0 (in-situ): This stage of cancer is in the top lining of the lung or bronchus. It hasn't spread to other parts of the lung or outside of the lung.

Stage I: This cancer hasn't spread outside the lung.

Stage II: This Cancer is larger than Stage I, has spread to lymph nodes inside the lung, or there's more than one tumor in the same lobe of the lung.

Stage III: Cancer is larger than Stage II, has spread to nearby lymph nodes or structures or there's more than one tumor in a different lobe of the same lung.

Stage IV: Cancer has spread to the other lung, the fluid around the lung, the fluid around the heart or distant organs.

Limited VS. Extensive Stage

While providers now use stages I through IV for small cell lung cancer, you might also hear it described as a limited or extensive stage. This is based on whether the area can be treated with a single radiation field.

Limited stage SCLC is confined to one lung and can sometimes be in the lymph nodes in the middle of the chest or above the collar bone on the same side.

Extensive stage SCLC is widespread throughout one lung or has spread to the other lung, lymph nodes on the opposite side of the lung, or to other parts of the body.

1.2 Causes and Risk Factors

Anyone can get lung cancer. Lung cancer happens when cells in the lung mutate or change. Various factors can cause this mutation (a permanent change in the DNA sequence of a gene) to happen. Most often, this change in lung cells happens when people breathe in dangerous, toxic substances. Even if you were exposed to these substances many years ago, you are still at risk for lung cancer. Talk to your doctor if you have been exposed to any of the substances listed below and take steps to reduce your risk and protect your lungs. The following are the causes of lung cancer:

Smoking: Smoking is the number one cause of lung cancer. It causes about 90 percent of lung cancer cases. Tobacco smoke contains many chemicals that are known to cause lung cancer. If you still smoke, quitting smoking is the single best thing you can do for your lung health. Smokers are not the only ones affected by cigarette smoke. If you are a former smoker, your risk is decreased, but has not gone away completely—you can still get lung cancer.

Nonsmokers also can be affected by smoking. Breathing in secondhand smoke puts you at risk for lung cancer or other illnesses.

Radon: Radon exposure is the second-leading cause of lung cancer. Radon is a colorless, odorless radioactive gas that exists naturally in soil. It comes up through the soil and enters buildings through small gaps and cracks. One out of every 15 homes in the U.S. is subject to radon exposure. Exposure to radon combined with cigarette smoking seriously increases your lung cancer risk.

Hazardous Chemicals: Exposure to certain hazardous chemicals poses a lung cancer risk. Working with materials such as asbestos, uranium, arsenic, cadmium, chromium, nickel and some petroleum products is especially dangerous. If you think you may be breathing in hazardous chemicals at your job, talk to your employer and your doctor to find out to protect yourself.

Particle Solution: Particle pollution refers to a mix of very tiny solid and liquid particles that are in the air we breathe. Evidence shows that particle pollution—like that coming from that exhaust smoke—increases the risk of lung cancer.

Gene: Genetic factors also may play a role in one's chances of developing lung cancer. A family history of lung cancer may mean you are at a higher risk of getting the disease. If others in your family have or ever had lung cancer, it's important to mention this to your doctor.

1.3 Common Symptoms and Diagnosis

Different people have different symptoms for lung cancer. Some people have symptoms related to the lungs. Some people whose lung cancer has spread to other parts of the body (metastasized) have symptoms specific to that part of the body. Some people just have general symptoms of not feeling well. Most people with lung cancer don't have symptoms until the cancer is advanced. Lung cancer symptoms may include:

- Coughing that gets worse or doesn't go away.
- Chest pain.
- Shortness of breath.
- Wheezing.
- Coughing up blood.
- Feeling very tired all the time.

- Weight loss with no known cause.

Other changes that can sometimes occur with lung cancer may include repeated bouts of pneumonia and swollen or enlarged lymph nodes (glands) inside the chest in the area between the lungs.

These signs and symptoms can happen with other illnesses, too. If you have some of these signs and symptoms, talk to your doctor, who can help find the cause.

Now, How is Lung Cancer Diagnosed?

Lung cancer is diagnosed through imaging tools, including computed tomography (CT), magnetic resonance imaging (MRI) and positron emission tomography (PET) scans.

Once a doctor determines that there is reason to suspect that there may be cancer, he or she may use additional testing, including a biopsy, ultrasound, mediastinoscopy, thoracoscopy or wedge resection.

It is a complex disease, with a number of causes, several types of tumors and various symptoms, which means that an accurate diagnosis is critical for the best possible prognosis. A medical center with experience in diagnosing and treating lung cancer is more likely to accurately diagnose the cause of symptoms.

The imaging tools includes:
CT scans, which use X-rays to create cross-sectional images of the chest.

MRI scans, which use radio waves and strong magnets to create detailed images of soft tissue. Like CT scans, they can produce detailed images of the tissue in the chest cavity. They are most often used to see if lung cancer has spread beyond its initial site.

PET scans, which use fluorodeoxyglucose (FDG) injected into the body to illuminate cancer cells. It's also useful in determining if cancer has spread beyond the initial site.

PET/CT scans, which combine the technology of both to give the doctor an even more detailed image.

Once a doctor determines that there is reason to suspect that there may be cancer (or some other condition), he or she will order further testing, which may include one or more of the following procedures.

Biopsies, which are the most common tool to obtain tissue for diagnosing lung cancer. Depending on where the nodule is located and the patient's physical condition, the doctor will do either a needle biopsy or a bronchoscopy.

During a needle biopsy, the surgeon uses a syringe to remove tissue from the nodule. A CT scan guides the surgeon to the nodule. This type of test is usually done under sedation rather than under general anesthesia so that it can be done as an outpatient procedure without a hospital stay.

Bronchoscopy is a biopsy done by passing a tube called a bronchoscope through the patient's mouth or nose, down into the trachea (windpipe) and then into the lungs where the suspicious nodule is located. Tissue is then obtained via needle, which the patient does not feel, from the bronchoscope. Depending on whether a flexible or rigid bronchoscope is used, the procedure will be done under sedation or general anesthesia. The advantage of a bronchoscopy is that the surgeon can evaluate the airways at the same time. At Hopkins, surgeons have the option of using ultrasound-guided or navigational bronchoscopies. A navigational bronchoscopy uses electromagnetic technology to guide the bronchoscope.

Endobronchial ultrasound (EBUS) is a kind of bronchoscopy with an ultrasound probe that can send sound waves throughout the chest cavity, allowing doctors to look at the area on an ultrasound monitor. The doctor can then take tissue samples from a nodule or other areas that may look suspicious.

Mediastinoscopy is a surgical procedure that requires general anesthesia. An incision is made in the neck so that a lighted instrument called a mediastinoscope can be inserted to examine the area between the lungs known as the mediastinum. Biopsies of the mediastinal lymph nodes are taken for cancer staging.

Video-assisted thoracoscopy (VAT) allows the doctor to see where the nodule is located, as well as the surrounding area. For this diagnostic procedure, a tiny camera is inserted through the airway on a thin, tube-like instrument. Using surgical instruments, the surgeon can remove as much tissue as is necessary for testing. A pathologist can test the nodule while the patient is still under anesthesia so that the surgeon can clear the section around the nodule if it is cancerous.

Wedge resection is surgery used to remove a triangular section of tissue, including a nodule or tumor. It may be used as a diagnostic procedure to determine if a suspicious nodule is cancerous. A wedge resection removes the smallest possible amount of tissue. If tissue is found to be cancerous on a wedge resection, additional surgery may be required.

1.4 Statistics and Prognosis

Worldwide, lung cancer is the second most commonly diagnosed cancer. NSCLC is the most common type of lung cancer in the United States, accounting for 81% of all lung cancer diagnoses.

In 2023, an estimated 238,340 adults (117,550 men and 120,790 women) in the United States will be diagnosed with lung cancer. Worldwide, an estimated 2,206,771 people were diagnosed with lung cancer in 2020. These statistics include both small cell lung cancer and NSCLC.

Since around 2006, incidence rates in the United States have dropped over 1% each year in women compared to 2.6% each year in men. The drop in cases for both men and women are due to fewer people smoking.

Currently, Black and White women have lower incidence rates than men. Black men, who have the highest lung cancer rates, are about 12% more likely to get lung cancer than White men. Black women are 16% less likely to get lung cancer when compared with White women.

The risk of lung cancer increases with age. An estimated 53% of all people diagnosed with the disease are age 70 or older. An estimated 83% of cases are diagnosed in people aged 65 or older. Men are most likely to be diagnosed with NSCLC between the ages of 80 and 84, while most cases in women are found between the ages of 75 and 79.

Lung cancer is the leading cause of cancer death for men and women worldwide. It is estimated that 127,070 deaths (67,160 men and 59,910 women) from this disease will occur in the United States in 2023. In 2020, an estimated 1,796,144 people died worldwide from the disease.

Lung cancer makes up around 20% of cancer deaths in the United States. However, death rates for the disease through 2020 have declined by 58% since 1990 in men and 36% since 2002 in women. From 2014 to 2020, the death rates for men with lung cancer dropped by around 5% each year. The death rates for women with lung cancer declined 4% per year during the same period. Research suggests that these declines are due to fewer people starting smoking, more people quitting smoking, and advances in diagnosis and treatment.

Since 1990, Black men have experienced the largest declines in death rate for lung cancer among men. In the early 1990s, Black men were 40% more likely to die from the disease than White men, compared to 14% during 2016 to 2020. Among women, Black women saw the sharpest drop in death rate since the early or late 2000s. In 2020, the lung cancer death rate in

Black women was 17% lower than White women, compared to 4% in 1990.

What is the Survival Rate?

There are different types of statistics that can help doctors evaluate a person's chance of recovery from NSCLC. These are called survival statistics. A specific type of survival statistic is called the relative survival rate. It is often used to predict how having cancer may affect life expectancy. Relative survival rate looks at how likely people with NSCLC are to survive for a certain amount of time after their initial diagnosis or start of treatment compared to the expected survival of similar people without this cancer.

It is important to remember that statistics on the survival rates for people with NSCLC are only an estimate. They cannot tell an individual person if cancer will or will not shorten their life. Instead, these statistics describe trends in groups of people previously diagnosed with the same disease, including specific stages of the disease.

The 5-year relative survival rate for all types of lung cancer in the United States is 23%. For NSCLC, the 5-year relative survival rate is 28%.

The survival rates for lung cancer vary based on several factors. These include the stage of cancer, a person's age and general health, and how well the treatment plan works. Another factor that can affect outcomes is the subtype of lung cancer.

The 5-year relative survival rate for NSCLC in women in the United States is 33%. The 5-year relative survival rate for men is 23%.

For people with localized NSCLC, which means the cancer has not spread outside the lung, the overall 5-year relative survival rate is 65%. However, around 70% of people with NSCLC are diagnosed after the cancer has spread outside the lung. For regional NSCLC, which means the cancer has spread outside of the lung to nearby lymph nodes, the 5-year relative survival rate is about 37%. When cancer has spread to distant parts of the body, called metastatic lung cancer, the 5-year relative survival rate is 9%. It is important to note that newer treatments like targeted therapies and immunotherapies are allowing people with metastatic lung cancer to live longer than ever before.

Each year, tens of thousands of people are cured of NSCLC in the United States. In 2022, there were more than 650,000 people alive in the United States who have a history of lung cancer. And, some patients with advanced lung cancer can live many years after diagnosis. Sometimes patients who are told that their lung cancer is incurable live longer than many who are told that their lung cancer is curable. The important thing to remember is that lung cancer is treatable at any stage, and these treatments have been proven to help people with lung cancer live longer with better quality of life.

Experts measure relative survival rate statistics for NSCLC every 5 years. This means the estimate may not reflect the results of advancements in how NSCLC is diagnosed or treated from the last 5 years. Talk with your doctor if you have any questions about this information.

Chapter 2: Coping With the Diagnosis

2.1 Emotional Impact

It is completely normal to worry. People with a cancer diagnosis often feel their world is turned upside-down, because it often is, and not just at the time of diagnosis. Allow yourself to mourn the loss of what you expected your life to be, or what you think it should be or will be. Work toward finding peace with what it is and how you can not only survive, but thrive. Coping with illness can feel like a full-time job, and anyone who has been through treatment knows it can take a psychological toll.

Here's what you can do:

- Talk about it by sharing with friends and family about how you're feeling, seek peer support through groups like the Lung Cancer Survivors Community on Inspire and find a therapist who has experience working with clients who are experiencing life-limiting illness.

- Identify what is within your control. The easiest way to do this is by educating yourself. Ask your medical team questions, even if you find yourself asking the same ones over and over again. Living with cancer can be overwhelming, and when we're overwhelmed, it's harder to process and retain information. Educate yourself on your diagnosis and treatment options, and know that you can always make adjustments down the line. Your treatment decisions are within your control.

- Keep an open dialogue with your medical team as well as your support system. Have honest discussions with your loved ones and healthcare providers not only about how you're feeling but also your quality of life goals. Focus on your goals, especially on bad days.

2.2 Seeking Support

Being able to speak freely within a trusted and supporting group can positively impact your health. Find the type of support group that is right for you.

Online Support Community: The American Lung Association has a free online lung cancer community on Inspire.com called Lung Cancer Survivors for individuals who are living with lung diseases and their caregivers. Individuals register to join the community. Members can choose their level of participation and engagement. This online lung cancer forum is a place for members to discuss how lung disease is affecting them and share their life experience with their peers.

Get a Mentor Angel or Become a Mentor Angel: There are groups created to match people with lung cancer, you can find one to seek support from people who have been in your shoes or become a mentor and offer support to someone facing the cancer.

Social Support: Social support groups such as Better Breathers Club that gives you the tools you need to live the best quality of life you can and also their meetings are in person, Patient and Caregiver Network, which is a nationwide, online patient support program providing direct access to education, support and connection to others also living with lung disease.

2.3 Second Opinions and Treatment Planning

Finding the right medical care is important. You should feel comfortable with your doctor and confident you are receiving the best care possible. You have the right to seek a second (or third or fourth) opinion about your lung cancer treatment plan. Below are some signs that a second opinion could be helpful.

You Aren't Being Cared for by Specialists: It is important for a physician or group of physicians who specialize in lung cancer to review your case and treatment plan. Professionals who specialize in lung cancer like thoracic oncologists are the most up-to-date on lung cancer treatment guidelines and emerging treatments. There may not be a specialist at the hospital where you are being treated. In that case, you might want to seek a second opinion at a large hospital, like one affiliated with a university or large medical institution. Or your doctor may be able to share your case with specialists at another hospital for input.

Your Doctor Makes You Feel to Blame for Your Cancer: No one deserves lung cancer. No matter what your health history is, you are not to blame for your cancer. If you feel like your doctor lacks compassion, it is time to seek a second opinion.

Your Doctor Gets Upset When You Ask Questions: The best relationship between a doctor and a patient is a collaborative one. It is important to feel comfortable asking questions and feel satisfied with the answers. Read up on as much information as you can and find a doctor who wants to have conversations with you about your care.

Your Doctor Tells You There is Nothing to be Done and to "Get Your Affairs in Order": The subject of prognosis is a tough one. Your treatment decisions should be made after careful consideration and conversations with your care team. While the lung cancer survival rate isn't where we would like it to be, progress is being made every day and treatment options are expanding. If you feel your doctor is dismissing your case and not giving you hope, it may be time to seek a second opinion.

Your Doctor Doesn't Know What Biomarker Testing is or Refuses to Talk to You About It: Biomarker testing looks for specific markers on your tumor, sometimes called molecular or genomic markers. The results from this testing help inform your possible treatment options such as whether to take a targeted therapy or participate in a clinical trial. This type of testing is especially important for patients with non-small cell lung cancer, who are most likely to have these markers. If your doctor is unable or unwilling to discuss biomarker testing, it may be time to seek a second opinion.

Chapter 3: Treatment Options

3.1 Surgery, Radiotherapy and Chemotherapy

Surgery

There are 3 main types of lung cancer surgery:

- lobectomy – where 1 of the large parts of the lung (lobes) is removed. Your doctors will suggest this operation if the cancer is just in 1 section of 1 lung.

- pneumonectomy – where the entire lung is removed. This is used when the cancer is located in the middle of the lung or has spread throughout the lung.

- wedge resection or segmentectomy – where a small piece of the lung is removed. This procedure is only suitable for a small number of patients. It is only used if your doctors think your cancer is small and limited to one area of the lung. This is usually very early-stage non-small-cell lung cancer. You may be concerned about being able to breathe if some or all of your lung is removed, but it's possible to breathe normally with 1 lung.

However, if you have breathing problems before the operation, it's likely these symptoms will continue after surgery.

Radiotherapy

Radiotherapy uses pulses of radiation to destroy cancer cells. There are a number of ways it can be used to treat lung cancer.

- An intensive course of radiotherapy, known as radical radiotherapy, may be used to treat non-small-cell lung cancer if you are not healthy enough for surgery.

- For very small tumours, a special type of radiotherapy called stereotactic radiotherapy may be used instead of surgery.

- Radiotherapy can also be used to control the symptoms, such as pain and coughing up blood, and to slow the spread of cancer when a cure is not possible (this is known as palliative radiotherapy).

- A type of radiotherapy known as prophylactic cranial irradiation (PCI) is also sometimes used during the treatment of small-cell lung cancer. PCI involves treating the whole brain with a low dose of radiation. It's used as a preventative measure because there's a risk that small-cell lung cancer will spread to your brain.

Chemotherapy

Chemotherapy uses powerful cancer-killing medicine to treat cancer. There are several ways that chemotherapy can be used to treat lung cancer. For example, it can be:

- given before surgery to shrink a tumour, which can increase the chance of successful surgery (this is usually only done as part of a clinical trial).

- given after surgery to prevent the cancer returning

- used to relieve symptoms and slow the spread of cancer when a cure is not possible.

- combined with radiotherapy

Chemotherapy treatments are usually given in cycles. A cycle involves taking chemotherapy medicine for several days, then having a break for a few weeks to let the therapy work and for your body to recover from the effects of the treatment.

The number of cycles you need will depend on the type and grade of lung cancer. Most people need 4 to 6 cycles of treatment over 3 to 6 months.

You will see your doctor after these cycles have finished. If the cancer has improved, you may not need any more treatment.

If the cancer has not improved after these cycles, your doctor will tell you if you need a different type of chemotherapy. Alternatively, you may need maintenance chemotherapy to keep the cancer under control.

Chemotherapy for lung cancer involves taking a combination of different medicines. The medicines are usually given through a drip into a vein (intravenously), or into a tube connected to one of the blood vessels in your chest.

Some people may be given capsules or tablets to swallow instead.

Before you start chemotherapy, your doctor might prescribe you some vitamins and/or give you a vitamin injection.

These can help reduce some of the side effects.

3.2 Targeted Therapy and Immunotherapy

Targeted Therapy

Targeted therapies (also known as biological therapies) are medicines designed to slow the spread of advanced non-small cell lung cancer. Targeted therapies are only suitable for people who have certain proteins in their cancerous cells.

Your doctor may request tests on cells removed from your lung (a biopsy) to see if these treatments are suitable for you.

Immunotherapy

Immunotherapy is a group of medicines that stimulate your immune system to target and kill cancer cells. It can be used on its own or combined with chemotherapy. Some of the immunotherapy medicines used to treat lung cancer are pembrolizumab and atezolizumab.

You might have immunotherapy through a plastic tube that goes into:

- a large vein your chest (central line)

- a vein in your arm (cannula): It takes around 30 to 60 minutes to receive a dose, and you may need a dose every 2 to 4 weeks. If the side effects are not too difficult to manage and the therapy is successful, immunotherapy can be taken for up to 2 years.

3.3 Clinical Trials

Clinical trials are research studies that test new and promising treatments directly with patients.

In fact, today's gold standard treatment options were once studies in a clinical trial. These studies may also test new ways to prevent or diagnose diseases such as lung cancer. It may include new ways to take medicine, radiation therapy, or surgery. Clinical trial teams make sure you receive the safest and best care. If you are recently diagnosed, you do not need to wait to consider a clinical trial for your treatment. No matter where you are in your treatment process, a clinical trial could be a good option for you.

For some people, the thought of participating in a research study is uncomfortable. They may have trust issues about the treatment they will receive. They may worry about the ways they will feel included in the process.

Over time, researchers have learned many valuable lessons about the importance of trust. Decades ago, trial staff did not share the information participants needed to know about issues such as safety or goals. This was a serious issue for diverse communities and influences recruitment efforts to this day. As a result, the rules were changed to make sure everyone is given information but also ensure the information was understood.

Today, researchers design clinical trials to make certain that:

- Participants receive all the information they need through a process called Informed Consent before they agree to join the research effort.

- Trial staff strive to enhance diversity and remove barriers about issues including participation and access such as help with transportation or support services.

- Community representation is a priority. For the research to be most helpful, trials must include the patients who are more vulnerable to the health condition.

3.4 Managing Treatment Side Effects

There are many treatments for lung cancer and these medications or therapies can often bring side effects. Throughout your diagnosis, you may be recommended a range of different options. Understanding how to manage lung cancer treatment side effects is important to help you live well. These can include lowered blood counts that can result in reduced immunity, anemia or bleeding problems; nausea and vomiting; diarrhea or constipation. Side effects can also include skin conditions, loss of appetite, weight loss and fatigue. Most side effects can be managed with the support of your healthcare team.

Fatigue

A common side effect of many lung cancer treatments is fatigue. This can include feeling exhausted, sleepy, drowsy, confused or impatient. Fatigue can also cause irritability, sadness and reduced care in your appearance or sexual desire. While you'll often only experience fatigue for a short period while undergoing treatment, it can impact on your quality of life and overall well being. This is why you should discuss how to best manage this side effect with your healthcare team.

Tips for managing fatigue:

- Organize activities throughout the day with rests in between, rather than being constantly 'on-the-go'

- Eat a balanced diet and drink at least 1.5 liters of water per day to stay hydrated and increase energy

- Avoid caffeine where possible as it can make you jittery and irritable

- Lean on your support network if you need help with everyday tasks like shopping, childcare or driving.

Skin Conditions

Dry and itchy skin can be a common side effect of radiotherapy and targeted cancer therapies. Even mild cases of skin flare-ups can cause irritation. It's important to seek advice from your doctor if you experience this.

Tips for managing dry skin:

- Use a perfume and preservative free moisturizer that contains urea or sorbolene cream to hydrate the skin

- Avoid hot baths and long showers

- Use a natural detergent and colloidal oatmeal wash rather than chemical-heavy soaps

- Avoid sun exposure and apply sunscreen everyday (unless you are undergoing radiotherapy)

- Maintain hydration by drinking at least 1.5 litres of water per day

- Protect your skin from the cold and wind.

Tips for managing itchy skin:

- Apply cold compresses (an icepack wrapped in a towel)

- Keep nails short to avoid scratching and try to dab or wipe skin for relief

- Use an anti-itch cream or powder for relief

- For more serious itching talk to your doctor about whether other medication may be an option.

Weight Loss

Loss of appetite and nausea are also common side effects of lung cancer treatments and can result in weight changes. If nausea leads to vomiting, it is important to keep fluids up to remain hydrated. Your doctor can also prescribe anti-nausea medication to help. Loss of appetite and nausea can result in weight loss. Because of this, managing these side effects with the support of your healthcare team is important to help you stay well.

Tips for managing loss of appetite and nausea:

- Eat small and frequent meals as large meals can exacerbate nausea.

- Eat and chew slowly to support digestion

- Try eating simple foods like dry toast or crackers.

- If you can keep liquids down better than food, try enriching your drinks with honey, yogurt or other nutritional supplement to support weight gain

- Prepare and freeze food before undergoing treatment to ensure you have easily accessible meals ready while undergoing therapy

- When in doubt, talk to a dietician to support your nutritional needs.

Chapter 4: Integrative Approaches to Wellness

4.1 Nutrition and Diet

Since cancer treatment can lead to fluctuations in appetite and body weight, it's important to pay close attention to your diet. In addition to helping you maintain a healthy weight, eating a balanced diet during chemotherapy or radiation therapy can help manage treatment side effects, increase energy, increase muscle tone, preserve immune function and reduce inflammation.

The following are foods you should add to your diet:

Plant-based Proteins: Some of the best foods to eat during chemotherapy or other cancer treatments are plant-based proteins. They offer the highest levels of vitamins and minerals. This means eating lots of vegetables as well as beans, legumes, nuts and seeds. If you do eat animal proteins, choose lean options like chicken or fish.

Healthy Fats: Monounsaturated and polyunsaturated fats also have health benefits. Avocados, olive oil, grapeseed oil and walnuts are all high in omega-3 fatty acids, which help combat inflammation and improve cardiovascular health.

Healthy Carbs: When choosing carbohydrates, opt for foods that are minimally processed, like whole wheat, bran and oats. These have soluble fiber, which helps maintain good gut bacteria. Soluble fiber also promotes the production of short-chain fatty acids (SCFAs), which lend a hand to everything from metabolism to cellular repair.

Vitamins and Minerals: Vitamins and minerals help our bodies' enzymatic processes, which play a big role in boosting immune function and reducing inflammation. When possible, select foods fortified with vitamin D. These may include milk, orange juice, yogurt and some cereals.

4.2 Exercise and Physical Activity

When it comes to exercise and lung cancer, the goal is to find the right amount that helps you feel more energized but doesn't tire you out. Low-intensity activities, like easy walking, light stretching, gentle yoga, tai chi are great options for improving your cardiovascular health without overdoing it.

For easy walking, choose walking over driving when possible, or make it a habit to go for a short walk after dinner each night.

For light stretching, start and end the day with a few simple stretches to prevent muscle tightness and joint stiffness.

Gentle yoga, check out gentle yoga classes at studios in your community or online. Make sure to pick a class that's geared toward gentle, restorative yoga postures. An added benefit to yoga is that you'll learn deep breathing exercises to improve your lung capacity.

Tai Chi, this ancient Chinese form of exercise is referred to as "moving meditation" and helps with focus, concentration, balance and mindfulness.

4.3 Managing Stress and Mindfulness

A lung cancer diagnosis can be emotionally overwhelming. The fear, anxiety, and uncertainty that often accompany the diagnosis can create immense stress. Furthermore, the physical discomfort and distressing side effects of treatments like chemotherapy and radiation therapy can exacerbate this stress. The necessary lifestyle changes, including alterations to diet, exercise, and work schedules, can add further complexity. Therefore, stress management is crucial for individuals living with lung cancer.

To effectively manage stress in the context of lung cancer, it's essential to adopt various strategies. Firstly, educating oneself about the condition and its treatments can reduce anxiety by increasing awareness. Secondly, open communication with healthcare teams, friends, and family provides essential support. Practices like mindfulness meditation, exercise, and maintaining a healthy diet can significantly reduce stress. Seeking professional counseling and joining support groups are also valuable resources for emotional support and coping strategies.

Mindfulness, the practice of being fully present in the moment without judgment, is a powerful tool for individuals with lung cancer. It offers various benefits, including stress reduction, improved pain management, enhanced emotional well-being, and better coping with the challenges of a lung cancer diagnosis and treatment. Also, it helps individuals become more in tune with their bodies and emotions, fostering a sense of control and resilience during a difficult journey.

Incorporating mindfulness into one's daily routine can be transformative. Dedicate a few minutes each day to mindfulness exercises, such as meditation or deep breathing. Practice mindful eating, paying attention to the sensations of eating and how it makes you feel. Engage in activities like yoga or Tai Chi that incorporate mindfulness and gentle movement. Lastly, practice self-compassion by being kind to yourself and acknowledging that experiencing a wide range of emotions during your lung cancer journey is entirely normal. Combining these stress management techniques with mindfulness can significantly improve the well-being and quality of life for individuals facing a lung cancer diagnosis, creating a more positive and fulfilling experience.

4.4 Complementary and Alternative therapies

Complementary therapies may help to control your symptoms and enhance your quality of life. They may be used alongside conventional cancer treatments. This therapy works using the healing power of nature, stimulating the body's natural healing ability.

There is a huge variety of complementary therapies advertised on the open market. Many are well known and proven to be helpful. However, there are also some therapies that have doubtful or unproven benefits. It is important to also check with your doctor before starting any complementary therapy as it may interfere with some treatments or other medication you may be taking.

There are so many tykes of complementary therapies one could go for. There are:
Acupuncture, aromatherapy, bowen technique, hypnotherapy, massage, reflexology, reiki, spiritual healing, tai chi.

It is important to stress that there is no conclusive scientific proof that such treatments can reduce (shrink) or cure cancer.

You should also be very wary of unusual (possibly illegal) and often costly therapies advertised in the media such as the internet, or newspaper adverts, including cannabis oil. Trust information from reputable sources and be wary of links shared on social networks claiming miracle cures.

If you are in any doubt, speak to your GP or hospital team about whether it may be of any benefit to you. They may even have a complementary therapy service they can refer you to.

Chapter 5: Living a Fulfilling Life

5.1 Balancing Life and Cancer

Treating non-small cell lung cancer (NSCLC) is a process that can take many months or years. During that time, you may go through chemotherapy cycles, radiation treatments, surgery, and many doctor's appointments.

NSCLC treatment can be exhausting and time-consuming, so it's important to find some balance. Here are some tips to help you get the most out of life while you're treating your cancer.

Relieve Your Symptoms: Both lung cancer and its treatments can cause side effects like fatigue, nausea, weight loss, and pain. It's hard to get enjoyment out of life when you don't feel well.

But there are ways to manage your side effects. A group of treatments collectively known as palliative care can relieve your side effects and help you feel better. You can get palliative care from the doctor who treats your cancer, or at a center that provides this type of care.

Put Work on Hold: About 46 percent of cancer survivors in the United States are of working age, and many older adults are continuing to work past age 64. A job can sometimes be a positive thing, taking your mind off the stresses of treatment. Yet having to go to work when you don't feel well can also add to your stress.

You may need extra time off to focus on your treatment and to give your body time to recover. Ask your human resources department for your company's policy on paid and unpaid leave, and how long you can take off. If your company doesn't offer you time off, check whether you qualify under the Family Medical Leave Act (FMLA) or other federal or state programs.

Adjust Your Priorities: Before NSCLC, your life might have followed a set routine. Cancer can throw you off your normal schedule.

There may be things you need to put on hold right now — like cleaning your house or cooking for your family. Do only as much as you can. Delegate less critical tasks to the people around you so you can focus all your energy on healing.

Relax: When you feel overwhelmed, take a few deep breaths. Meditation — a practice that combines breathing with mental focus — helps to relieve stress and improve the quality of life in people with lung cancer.

Yoga and massage are two other relaxation techniques that calm both your mind and body. Everyday activities can be relaxing, too. Listen to your favorite songs. Take a warm bath. Or, play catch with your kids.

Do What You Love: Cancer treatment takes a lot of time and energy. But you can still find time to enjoy simple activities. Though you might not have the energy for activities like rock climbing or mountain biking, you can still do at least some of the things you love.

See a Funny Movie With a Friend. Curl up with a good book. Walk outside for a few minutes to clear your mind. Take up a hobby like scrapbooking or knitting.

Eat Well: Chemotherapy and other cancer treatments can reduce your appetite and change the way foods taste. A lack of desire to eat can prevent you from getting the nutrients you need.

During cancer treatment is one time when you don't need to count calories. Eat the foods you love, and that taste good to you. Also, keep your favorite snacks on hand. Sometimes it's easier to eat small portions throughout the day, rather than three big meals.

5.2 Work and Financial Considerations

Treatment for lung cancer can vary depending on the extent of your disease but may include radiation, surgery, or chemotherapy.

Since treatment can last for several weeks or months, you may be asking: Will I be able to work while undergoing treatment for lung cancer? And if so, how much should I work?

The ability to work during treatment for lung cancer varies from person to person. It's important to ask your doctor how your specific treatment could affect your career. Under certain circumstances, your doctor might suggest it's time to stop working or to not work certain jobs.

Lung cancer can cause symptoms like shortness of breath and coughing. Depending on the nature of your job, working could potentially compromise your lung health. For example, you might work in a restaurant, bar, or another place that allows indoor smoking. Or maybe you're exposed to chemicals on the job or you work in a poorly ventilated environment. Both scenarios can exacerbate your symptoms.

Your doctor might also recommend not working if your job is fast-paced, which could trigger extreme shortness of breath. Frequent moving around and too few breaks can also cause breathing issues.

If you must stop working, speak with your employer's HR department right away to discuss disability and unpaid leave options. If you're not eligible for disability through your employer, you can apply for Social Security disability insurance.

Consider other ways to manage your finances as you prepare to stop working. Do you have unused vacation time or personal leave? If you use this time and stop working, you might still receive a paycheck for a few weeks.

Also, consider whether you can live off of your savings account. Ask your lenders and creditors about hardship provisions. Some banks might defer your payments for a few months, or temporarily reduce your monthly payments if you're unable to work due to sickness. This can remove some financial burden while you're not working.

As a last resort, you can pull cash from your retirement account. Typically, you'll pay a penalty if you withdraw money from a 401(k) or an IRA before the age of 59 and a half. But, if your doctor confirms that you have a disability and can't work for at least a year, you're allowed to take money from your IRA penalty-free.

If you have a 401(k), ask your employer for a hardship withdrawal. Keep in mind that you'll pay regular income tax on these withdrawals.

5.3 Family and Relationships

People said that when they first told family members about their lung cancer they were usually met with expressions of shock, fear, and distress - some did not know how to react and seemed embarrassed. Relationships within families can change as the result of illness, and sometimes news of the diagnosis helped to bring family members closer together. Some patients became aware of how important they were to their family and friends. It was sometimes hard to predict how other people would react to the diagnosis. Most family members offered great support, but a few people complained that support had not been forthcoming when they needed it. Some people emphasized that their loved ones had to face a very difficult time too and needed support and reassurance themselves.

Many people said that their friends felt uncomfortable and avoided them once they knew about the cancer diagnosis. Some of those with lung cancer found that others would cross the road to avoid a conversation because they did not know what to say. They thought that their friends were either embarrassed by the situation, or that they did not want to confront the idea of death. It was also suggested that other people might think that lung cancer patients were to blame because they had smoked.

Other people, however, reported that friends had been marvelous, helping with shopping, offering lifts to the hospital, providing practical help and making normal conversation as usual.

A few people said that they wanted other people to treat them as they had treated them before the diagnosis. They didn't want others to react with tears. Others commented that they did not want fake sympathy.

Some people realized that the diagnosis and the illness had made them self-absorbed or short tempered.

One man said since his diagnosis of lung cancer his friends and family had reassessed their lives, their working conditions, and use of recreational drugs. A woman said that as soon as she told her friends that she was ill they had sent her flowers, and then rushed to their doctors for checks-ups, fearing they might be ill too.

In other words, your family and friends no matter who you are or what you are should be able to guide you through your cancer journey. No one should blame you for it.

5.4 Travel and Adventure

Before booking a trip, it is important for travelers with a respiratory condition to research their destination, as well as the journey, and carefully consider their itinerary. There may be limited health care capacity or expertise for managing respiratory complications, and triggers such as pollen, dust or heat, could be present in greater quantities. It may also not be possible to accommodate those with some specific requirements, for example there may be no reliable electricity for a CPAP machine. Travelers with pre-existing health conditions should book a pre-travel consultation with a healthcare professional at least four to six weeks before travel; it is then possible to discuss the specific health issues and support the traveler to plan carefully and have realistic expectations for a trip. An early appointment also offers the opportunity to check the traveler is up-to-date with all vaccines routinely recommended for those with a respiratory condition and check destination-specific advice.

It is important to ensure that the respiratory condition is well-controlled before travel, it may be necessary to have a check-up with the usual health care provider before the trip. Respiratory conditions, such as asthma, may deteriorate during travel. Travelers should have an up-to-date plan detailing what to do in an emergency, both in terms of self-management and when to seek urgent medical advice.

For some travelers it may be appropriate to carry rescue medication, such as antibiotics and/or steroids, to manage exacerbations, this decision should be based on a careful assessment with the traveler's usual health care provider.

Concerns about a person's fitness to fly because of a respiratory condition, or associated comorbidity, should be assessed before travel. Partial pressure of oxygen will decrease as the airplane reaches altitude and oxygen saturations of healthy travelers can fall to 85-91 percent. Most travelers will compensate for this. It is likely that travelers who can walk 50 meters at normal pace or climb one flight of stairs without severe dyspnoea (difficulty breathing) will tolerate a normal aircraft environment. However, some will require supplementary oxygen and an assessment will need to be made.

Airlines should be contacted prior to booking if supplementary oxygen or additional equipment, including nebulisers or CPAP machines, are required during travel. It is also important that before travel, travelers find out what help is available and if their needs and equipment requirements can be accommodated, any assistance required should be booked well in advance.

Chapter 6: Facing Challenges Head On

6.1 Recurrence and Advanced Cancer

Once a patient enters remission, they may believe that there is no more potential for lung cancer to return. However, remission is not the same thing as a cancer cure. Remission means that the signs and symptoms of the cancer have been reduced. Lung cancer recurrence happens when your cancer returns after you've been in remission for at least one year.

Your chances of lung cancer recurrence depend on which type you have and the stage of the lung cancer. The two main types of lung cancer are non-small-cell lung cancer (NSCLC) and small-cell lung cancer (SCLC).

Unfortunately, it is pretty likely for both types of lung cancer to return after treatment. NSCLC was found to have a 30-75% chance of recurrence in one study. SCLC is even more aggressive and holds an even higher chance of recurrence. Most people who undergo treatment for SCLC experience recurrence within a year or two of remission.

Lung cancer recurrence is most common within five years of diagnosis.
There are different types of lung cancer recurrence depending on where the cancer returns.

Local recurrence, local recurrence is when cancer returns to the lung close to where it was initially found.

Regional recurrence happens when cancer grows in the lymph nodes near the initial site.

Distant recurrence, occurs when the lung cancer is found in a new site far from where it was initially located, such as in the brain, bones, adrenal glands, or liver.

If lung cancer returns after at least one year of remission, your oncologist will tell you that you have recurring lung cancer. Recurring lung cancer is relatively common, and tests will be conducted to determine if the same type of cancer has returned or if you have secondary cancer.

In some cases, specific treatments can cause a secondary cancer to develop after the cancer has gone into remission. This is not the same as a recurrence and is referred to as a second cancer. If your doctor performs a biopsy and finds that the cancer cells look different, it is not a recurrence but a second type of cancer.

6.2 Palliative Care and End-of-Life Decisions

Palliative care is holistic care that is focused on helping patients with life-threatening or grave illnesses to achieve a better quality of life to the very end. It is aimed at averting or treating problems caused by the illness or its treatment, in the physical, emotional, social and spiritual spheres of the patient's life, even if there is no prospect of a cure. It may be termed "comfort care" because it aims at providing total support to the patient and the patient's family and managing symptoms throughout the course of the disease.

The goals of palliative/end-of-life (EOL) care may be summarized as:

- Alleviating physical suffering in order to ensure a higher quality of life.

- Giving spiritual, psychological and social support to both patient and family.

- Encouraging open communication with the patient

- Coordinating care from different angles

- Honoring the values and care preferences expressed by the patient

- Preparing for death without unnecessary suffering, while allowing the family and the patient to achieve closure

The people involved in palliative care work as a team, comprising physicians, nurses, social workers, dietitians and psychologists. Some may have chaplains as well. They come to understand the patient's personal problems and may recommend to the primary care physician, ways and means to reduce distress and pain for the patient. This kind of care is at a premium when the disease can no longer be cured.

Another approach is hospice care, which is generally opted for when a patient is not expected to live longer than 6 months. The hospice team often provides medical, emotional and spiritual support including pain management in the patient's own home or in a hospice.

Want to learn about living with and beating prostate and breast cancer? Click here for prostate and click here for breast cancer to get a copy of my book on amazon.

Away from this book, it would be really appreciated if you could create time to provide a review if you thought it was worthwhile as it would motivate me. Thanks.